What's in Your Food?
RECIPE FOR DISASTER

Trans Fats

Stephanie Watson

rosen publishing's
rosen central

New York

To my father, who has always been my champion and greatest fan

Published in 2008 by The Rosen Publishing Group, Inc.
29 East 21st Street, New York, NY 10010

First Edition

Library of Congress Cataloging-in-Publication Data

Watson, Stephanie.
Trans fats / Stephanie Watson.
    p. cm.—(What's in your food? Recipe for disaster)
Includes bibliographical references and index.
ISBN-13: 978-1-4042-1418-7 (library binding)
1. Trans fatty acids—Popular works. 2. Lipids in human nutrition—
Popular works. I. Title.
QP752.T63.W38 2008
612.3'97—dc22

2007037756

Manufactured in China

Contents

Introduction

Life today moves quite fast. By the time school ends, your day is probably just beginning. There's sports practice, music lessons, after-school clubs, homework, chores, and get-togethers with your friends. With that kind of packed schedule, who has the time to sit down and eat three square meals a day?

On the busiest days, it's easier to grab something on the go. Fortunately, the food industry has made it easy for people to eat quickly. You can go to a fast-food drive-through window and get a bag stuffed with burgers and french fries in less than ten minutes. You can grab a handful of cookies out of your kitchen cabinet in a matter of seconds.

Although these quick foods taste good and satisfy your hunger, did you know that they contain ingredients that are dangerous to your health? One type of substance that you'll find in processed and fast foods can

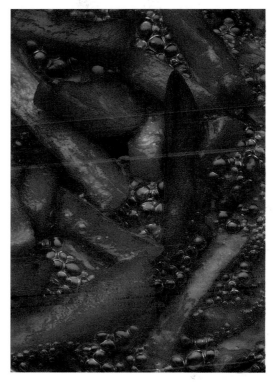

French fries get their crunch and rich flavor from trans fats. Although they may taste good, they're bad news for your arteries.

make you gain weight and raise your risk of becoming extremely sick. This substance is trans fat, and you can find it in some of your favorite foods, from french fries to breakfast cereal.

Restaurants and manufacturers use trans fats in their food to add taste and texture. Trans fats make fries crispy and delicious, give pies their flaky crust, and give doughnuts their rich, gooey feel. But while you're munching on fries, pies, and doughnuts, trans fats are making their way into your arteries and clogging them up. They're also adding inches to your waistline. They might even be taking years away from your life!

The Fattening of America

Health experts say that America is in the middle of an epidemic. It isn't a disease epidemic—it's a fat epidemic.

Two out of every three adults and one out of every five children are overweight, according to 2004 data from the Centers for Disease Control and Prevention (CDC).

All of that added weight is putting Americans at risk for serious health problems. One of the biggest problems is heart disease. It's the leading cause of death in the United States—more so than any other illness or injury. Almost half a million people died from heart disease in 2004, according to the American Heart Association.

Diabetes is a disease in which the body cannot produce an adequate amount of the hormone insulin. Type 2 of this disease is another major health problem linked to being overweight. When you're overweight, fat essentially covers your cells, making it difficult for your body to process insulin. The body uses insulin to convert sugar from foods into energy. Type 2 diabetes occurs when the body can't use insulin properly. Another form of diabetes, type 1, is not associated with being overweight. Type 1 diabetes is caused by a problem with the immune system.

In the past, almost all of the children who had diabetes had type 1. Today, because more and more young people are overweight, about half of all children who get diabetes have the type 2 kind. Here's a startling statistic from the CDC: out of every three children born in the United States in the year 2000, one is going to develop type 2 diabetes.

Why are so many American children overweight and unhealthy? Health experts say it's because they're eating more and moving less. Young people need to get

6

at least sixty minutes of exercise every day, according to the 2005 Dietary Guidelines from the U.S. Department of Agriculture. Research shows that young people aren't getting nearly that much. The President's Council on Physical Fitness and Sports finds that only 25 percent of high school students exercise for at least twenty minutes a day.

Part of the reason why young people aren't exercising is that they're spending more time in front of the television. On average, children watch more than three hours of television each day. Watching television cuts down on the time that they could actually be outside playing sports or otherwise exercising. It also makes children want to eat foods that aren't good for them because of all the tantalizing commercials.

If you're like most young people, you watch about forty thousand TV commercials every year, according to *The Handbook of Children and Media*. Most of those ads are for sugary cereal and candy, and for fattening fast foods. These commercials feature characters from your favorite movies and TV shows to tempt you into buying food that's not healthy for you.

Research shows that the ads are working. Young people are buying unhealthy food—lots of it. They're eating five times more fast food than they did in 1970, said Shanthy Bowman, Ph.D., and other researchers in a 2004 study. Every single day, one out of every three kids aged four to nineteen eats fast food. That fast food is loaded with extra salt, sugar, and fat—including trans fats.

7

You Are What You Eat

The old saying is true: You are what you eat. Fill up on fatty foods, and you're likely to become overweight and unhealthy. Eat plenty of fruits, vegetables, whole grains, and lean meats, and you'll keep your body feeling and looking its best.

The good news is that the word is spreading fast about healthy eating and its benefits. Food manufacturers and restaurants are getting wise to the dangers of trans fats and are starting to take them out of their foods. Foods that do contain trans fats now must say so on the label—the government requires it. Several cities are now forcing restaurants to get rid of all the trans fats on their menus.

Just because manufacturers are removing trans fats from their foods doesn't mean you're off the hook, though. You still need to make good choices about what you eat. In order to make good choices, you need to be an informed eater.

Don't get sucked in by pretty food packaging and slick TV commercials. Read before you eat. Food labels on packages and in many restaurants will tell you exactly how much total fat, trans fats, calories, sugar, and salt are in your food. Products that are too high in these unhealthy ingredients don't deserve a place on your plate.

Chapter One

Inside Fats

People tend to think of fat as the spongy white stuff around the edges of steak, or the soft stuff that jiggles around people's bellies and thighs. Actually, fat is the way in which animals and humans store energy. It comes from the foods you eat. Your body also makes some fat in your liver when your energy stores run low.

In scientific terms, fats are chemical compounds made from fatty acids. Each fatty acid is a chain consisting of hydrogen and carbon atoms. At one end of the chain is the group carbon-oxygen-oxygen-hydrogen (COOH). It's called a carboxyl group, and it's what puts the "acid" in fatty acids.

Just the Fats

Three types of fatty acids exist: saturated, monounsaturated, and polyunsaturated. Although all three fats share the same basic structure, their fatty acid chains are each a little bit different. Those small changes determine whether the fat is liquid or solid, and whether it is healthy or unhealthy.

Saturated fat is a solid, unhealthy kind of fat. On its chain, a hydrogen atom is attached to every single carbon atom. In other words, all of the carbon atoms are totally filled, or "saturated," with hydrogen atoms. All of the bonds that attach the atoms are single. (A single bond looks like this: C–C.)

Because the chains of saturated fats are so tightly packed, these fats tend to be solid at room temperature. Examples of saturated fats are red meat, cheese, and butter. These are the kinds of fats that raise the levels of an unhealthy fatlike substance called cholesterol in the blood and can lead to heart disease. A good rule of thumb is, the more solid the fat is at room temperature, the more harmful it is to you.

Unsaturated fat is often, but not always, a liquid and healthier type of fat. Fish, olive oil, and nuts contain unsaturated fats. On the fatty acid chain, unsaturated fats are missing some of the hydrogen atoms. The missing hydrogen atoms leave spaces, or gaps, in the chain. In places where there are missing hydrogen atoms, the carbon atoms are attached to each other by a double bond instead of a single bond. (A double bond looks like this: C = C.) Because of the gaps in the chain, unsaturated fatty acids are usually liquid at room temperature.

An unsaturated fatty acid that has just one double bond between carbon atoms is called monounsaturated.

("Mono" means "one.") A fatty acid that has more than one double bond between carbon atoms is called polyunsaturated. ("Poly" means "many.")

Unsaturated fatty acids come in two shapes: cis and trans. Whether or not a fat is cis or trans depends on where the hydrogen atoms sit on the carbon double bonds. Cis fatty acids have the hydrogen atoms on the same side of the chain. Trans fatty acids have hydrogen atoms on opposite sides of the chain. (*Trans* is Latin for "across.") Having all the hydrogen on the same side of the chain causes cis fatty acid chains to bend.

Although trans fats are unsaturated, their chains look more like saturated fats. Having less of a bend in

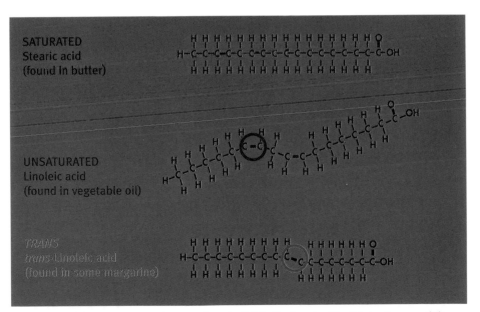

In saturated fats, every carbon molecule (C) is "saturated" with hydrogen (H) atoms. Unsaturated fats are missing a few hydrogen atoms. Trans fats are similar in structure to saturated fats.

the chain makes trans fats solid and more stable, which is why fast-food restaurants like to fry foods in them. Trans fats don't spoil as easily as cis fats do. The straighter chain also causes trans fats to be unhealthier by making them harder for people to digest. What's even scarier is that most trans fats are not found in nature. They're actually made by scientists in a laboratory!

Where Do Trans Fats Come From?

A very small amount of the trans fats people eat does come from natural sources, mainly meat and animal products. But a chemical process called hydrogenation produces the vast majority of trans fats in people's diets. Hydrogenation turns liquid vegetable oil into a more solid type of fat.

Hydrogenation starts out with natural materials, such as soybeans, corn, sunflower seeds, cottonseeds, and safflower seeds. These vegetable products are crushed to release their oils. Then, companies bubble hydrogen—a clear, odorless gas—through the vegetable oil at very high pressure and very high heat.

Hydrogenation saturates the fatty acid chain with hydrogen. Remember how in natural, unsaturated fatty acids, the hydrogen atoms were on the same side of the carbon chain? Hydrogenation moves some of the double bonds so that hydrogen atoms now sit on opposite sides of the chain. This makes the oil thicker and more solid, like the white paste you'll see if you open a jar of vegetable shortening.

Hydrogenation makes the oil more stable, so companies can fry foods in the same oil over and over again without it breaking down. It extends the shelf life of foods as well. This means that a box of cookies made with partially hydrogenated vegetable oil can sit on a supermarket shelf for months, even years, without spoiling.

Trans Fat Content in Some of Your Favorite Foods

The American Heart Association recommends limiting trans fats to about 2 grams or less *per day* . This list shows how many grams of trans fats you may be consuming in just *one serving* if you eat any of these popular foods.

Food	Total Fat	Trans Fat
Medium french fries	27 grams	8 grams
Doughnut	18 grams	5 grams
Pound cake (one slice)	16 grams	4–5 grams
Potato chips (small bag)	11 grams	3 grams
Stick margarine (one tablespoon)	11 grams	3 grams
Candy bar	10 grams	3 grams

Source: "Revealing Trans Fats." *FDA Consumer Magazine* (September–October 2003, Revised September 2005).

13

The History of Trans Fats

Today, food is plentiful. You can walk down a single city street and find literally dozens of restaurants and shops selling everything from pizza to ice cream to sandwiches. Back in the 1800s, though, that wasn't the case. People had to either grow their own food or work hard to earn the money to buy it.

In Europe during the 1800s, the working class could barely afford to buy animal products such as meat and butter. Without butter, it was hard for them to cook and bake. European governments became concerned that their people would go hungry.

In the 1860s, Emperor Napoléon III of France offered a prize to any scientist who could find a longer-lasting and

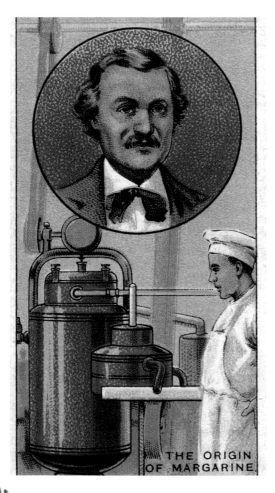

THE ORIGIN OF MARGARINE.

French scientist Hippolyte Mège-Mouriès invented margarine during the late 1860s.

cheaper alternative to butter. A French chemist named Hippolyte Mège-Mouriès took the challenge. He invented a butter substitute made from beef fat (tallow), water, and milk fat. He called it oleomargarine, after the fatty acid margaric acid.

In the early 1900s, scientists continued to work on the margarine formula. In 1902, German chemist Wilhelm Normann found that by adding hydrogen to vegetable oil, he could make a new, more solid kind of fat. The process he discovered was hydrogenation.

It wasn't long before partially hydrogenated oil made its way across the Atlantic Ocean to the United States. In 1911, the soap and candle company Procter & Gamble introduced its own partially hydrogenated vegetable shortening. It was called Crisco. The first Crisco advertisement, in 1912, claimed that the product would "affect every kitchen in America." It pretty much did. Americans loved Crisco's pure white look and the fact that it didn't spoil easily. Millions of people used it to bake, fry, and cook.

Then, a few other things happened that made partially hydrogenated vegetable oil even more popular. During World War II, butter was rationed, so Americans needed to use another product for frying and baking. Margarine seemed to be just the thing. It was cheap to cook with and tasted good.

Eating establishments picked up on partially hydro-genated oil, especially the new fast-food restaurants such as McDonald's, which were popping up everywhere from big cities to small towns. Partially hydrogenated oil worked perfectly for frying and baking. This oil was cheap and long lasting, and it made french fries and pies taste rich and delicious.

Food companies, too, liked partially hydrogenated oil. In the 1950s, a new system of roads crisscrossed the United States. These new roads allowed companies to ship their foods more easily across the country. Adding partially hydrogenated oil to pies, muffins, and other packaged foods meant that these foods could arrive in supermarkets in Chicago or Los Angeles just as fresh as they were when they left New York.

Not as Healthy as They Thought

In the 1970s, just about everyone was jumping on the margarine bandwagon. Studies came out linking saturated fat to high cholesterol and heart disease. People abandoned butter in favor of what they thought was healthier, vegetable-based margarine. At the same time, though, a small group of scientists was beginning to find that partially hydrogenated vegetable oil was even unhealthier than the animal fats it had replaced.

Yet, it wasn't until the 1990s that people began to really catch on about the dangers of trans fats. Many studies began linking trans fats to heart disease and death. In 1994, the Center for Science in the Public Interest (CSPI) was so worried about the threat of trans fats that it asked the U.S. Food and Drug Administration (FDA) to start requiring companies to list trans fats on food nutrition labels.

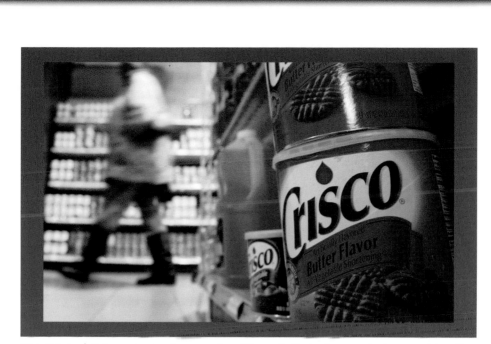

The original Crisco shortenIng, made with partially hydrogenated vegetable oil, was loaded with trans fats. The manufacturer has recently introduced a new version of Crisco with zero grams of trans fat per serving.

It took more than a decade for the FDA to adopt the rule. When it finally went into effect in January 2006, all companies had to start listing trans fats on their food labels. That same year, the New York City Department of Health ordered 20,000 restaurants in the city to stop using trans fats by the year 2008. The war against trans fats was officially under way.

Chapter Two

The Truth About Trans Fats

Fats are often portrayed as food demons in magazines and on TV news programs, but not all fats are evil. Some are actually good for your body when they're eaten in moderation. They give you energy. They make you feel full and satisfied after a meal. They help you absorb vitamins A, D, E, and K from the foods that you eat. They insulate your body from the cold and keep your skin and hair looking and feeling healthy. You need to include fats in your diet every day. You just want to include the good fats and skip the bad fats.

Examples of good fats are the omega-3 polyunsaturated fatty acids found in salmon, lake trout, mackerel, albacore tuna, sardines, and other fish. The American Heart Association says you should eat these fish at least twice per week because research shows they can actually protect against heart disease.

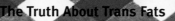

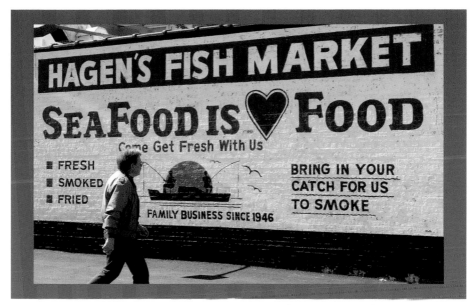

Research is showing that eating fish at least twice each week is good for your heart.

The real enemies to your body are saturated and trans fats. In large quantities, these types of fats can cause you to gain weight and become very sick. Here are just a few of the health problems that are linked to saturated and trans fats:

- **Obesity**. Fat packs a lot of calories. Each gram of fat contains 9 calories—more than double the 4 calories found in each gram of protein or carbohydrates. That's why you'll gain more weight eating a high-fat diet than you would eating a low-fat diet. Being overweight puts you at risk for all the following diseases.

- **Heart disease**. High-fat diets are rich in a fatlike substance called cholesterol. Although your body needs cholesterol in small amounts, too much of it can build up and form deposits called plaque on the inside of your arteries. Over time, these deposits can block the flow of blood throughout your body. If one of the deposits breaks free, it can form a clot that becomes lodged in the brain (called a stroke) or in an artery leading to the heart (called a heart attack).

- **Type 2 diabetes.** When you're overweight, your body has more trouble using insulin, a hormone that controls the amount of sugar in your blood. The inability of your body to adequately process insulin is called type 2 diabetes.

- **Cancer.** Normally, cells grow when they are needed and then they stop growing. In people with cancer, cells grow uncontrollably until they form masses called tumors. Cancerous tumors can spread throughout the body and damage organs. Studies have linked high-fat diets and obesity to several types of cancers, including those of the breast, colon, esophagus, and kidneys.

- **Asthma**. Studies have found that overweight people are much more likely to get asthma than people of average weight. Asthma causes the airways to become narrowed or blocked, making it difficult to breathe. Overweight people also have more trouble breathing and getting oxygen into their lungs while they sleep—a condition called sleep apnea.

What's in Your Chicken Nuggets?

Buy chicken nuggets and a large order of french fries at a fast-food restaurant in the United States, and your meal will be packed with far more trans fats than you would find in the same food order at a fast-food restaurant in Denmark. That's what Danish researchers Steen Stender, Jørn Dyerberg, and Arne Astrup found when they sampled french fries and chicken nuggets at McDonald's and Kentucky Fried Chicken restaurants in twenty different countries.

In the United States, a large order of fries and nuggets contained 10 grams of trans fats. In Hungary, that same order contained 25 grams of trans fats. But in Denmark, where the government limits the amount of trans fats that restaurants can use, each order contained less than 1 gram of the unhealthy fat. Because studies have found that even 5 grams per day of trans fats can increase the risk of heart disease by 25 percent, not only *what* you eat but also *where* you eat can make a big difference to your health.

Banning Trans Fats

The move to get trans fats out of people's diets is on, and it's being led by health experts and government officials. Denmark paved the way in 2004, when it banned foods containing oils made with more than 2 percent trans fats. The country switched to healthier oils containing cis unsaturated fatty acids.

Then, the New York City Board of Health voted to ban most trans fats from the city's 20,000 restaurants and 14,000 food suppliers. In 2007, Philadelphia,

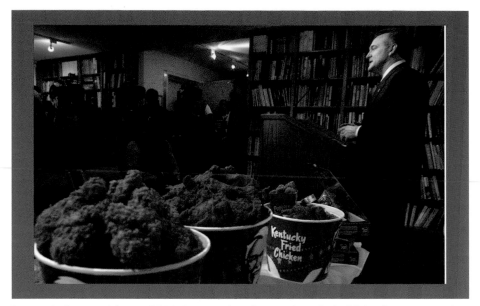

In 2006, the president of KFC Corporation (Kentucky Fried Chicken) announced that the company was switching to a cooking oil containing zero grams of trans fat.

Pennsylvania, and Montgomery County, Maryland, passed similar bans. Other locales are considering following their lead. As of January 1, 2006, the FDA requires all food manufacturers selling their products in the United States to list trans fats on the "Nutrition Facts" section of their labels.

Many restaurants and food manufacturers are responding to the fight against trans fats by removing it from their foods. In 2002, McDonald's promised to switch from its trans fat–filled oil to a healthier kind of oil. In April 2007, Kentucky Fried Chicken (KFC) announced that it had stopped frying chicken in trans fat–laden oil in all of its restaurants. Other restaurant chains, such as Wendy's, Panera Bread, California Pizza Kitchen, and Ruby Tuesday, have also switched to healthier oils.

These are all important steps in the right direction, but they don't mean that restaurants and packaged foods are now trans fat–free. As of 2007, McDonald's still had not replaced its unhealthy oils. Some of the restaurants, like KFC, which did stop using partially hydrogenated vegetable oils for frying, continued to use it as an ingredient in many of their other menu items.

The problem with getting the trans fat out of food is maintaining the same flavor and texture. Restaurants still want their french fries to taste as crispy and rich as they do when they're cooked in partially hydrogenated vegetable oils.

To make their foods seem healthier, some restaurants and food companies have left in the trans fats, but they've cut portion sizes to make it appear as though there is less trans fat in their food. Others have switched to butter, which is free of trans fats but is heavy in saturated fats. The search continues for the perfect, healthy fat.

Chapter Three

What Trans Fats Do to Your Body

To get an idea of just how dangerous trans fats are to the body, consider this: if Americans cut most of the artificial trans fats from their diets, between 72,000 and 228,000 fewer people would have heart attacks and die from heart disease *each year*. That's according to a 2006 study by Dariush Mozaffarian and other researchers.

Trans fats are so deadly because of what they do to arteries, the tubes that transport blood throughout the body. Like saturated fats, trans fats raise levels of low-density lipoprotein (LDL) cholesterol. This is the "bad" type of cholesterol that clogs arteries and prevents blood from flowing through. If blood gets stuck in an artery behind a big clog, the heart can literally starve, leading to heart disease and a life-threatening heart attack.

Trans fats are a double whammy. Not only do they *raise* bad LDL cholesterol, but

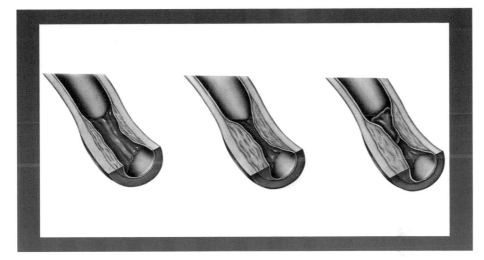

This illustration shows fatty cholesterol building up in arteries and eventually *(far right)* blocking blood flow to the heart.

they also *lower* the "good" high-density lipoprotein (HDL) cholesterol. When there is too much cholesterol in the blood, HDL cholesterol cleans up the excess and carries it to the liver so that it can be removed from the body. It helps keep arteries open by acting as the body's own drain cleaner.

Actually, trans fats are a *quadruple* whammy. They also raise levels of triglycerides, a form of fat in the blood, and they increase the amount of lipoprotein (a), a substance made up of protein and fat that transports cholesterol in the blood. These substances are hard on arteries. Excess triglycerides and lipoprotein (a) make healthy, flexible arteries turn hard and stiff. People with hard arteries are much more likely to have a heart attack or stroke.

Myths & Facts

Myth: Margarine is healthier than butter.

Myth: If a food package is labeled "0 Grams Trans Fat," it means that food contains no trans fat.

Myth: If I stop eating trans fats, I'll be healthier and I'll lose weight.

The Evidence

Researchers aren't just guessing when they say that trans fats cause all of these problems in the body. They have studies, made up of thousands of people, which show the real-life effects of consuming trans fats. One example is the 1993 Nurses' Health Study, which included eighty-five thousand women. The women in this study who ate the most trans fats were 50 percent more likely to have a heart attack than women who

Chunky Monkeys

Monkeys are known for being partial to bananas and other fruits. Scientists wanted to find out what would happen if they gave our simian friends a more human type of diet. Researchers at Wake Forest University used as their subjects two groups of green monkeys. They fed one group an American-style diet with about 8 percent of the fats coming from trans fats. They fed the other group a diet made up mostly of monounsaturated fats (such as olive oil) and no trans fats.

After six years, both groups of monkeys had gained weight, the researchers reported at a 2006 American Diabetes Association meeting. The chunkiest monkeys, though, were the ones that had eaten trans fats. Their weight had increased by 7.2 percent, compared with only a 1.8 percent weight increase in the other group. Most of the trans fat–fed monkeys gained weight in their belly, the most dangerous kind of fat. After eating trans fats for so many years, the monkeys' bodies no longer responded as well to insulin, which meant that they were at risk for type 2 diabetes.

27

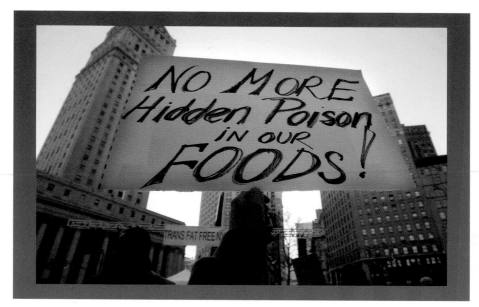

In 2006, people rallied against trans fats in New York City. That same year, the city's board of health voted to ban the dangerous fats from restaurants.

ate the least amount of trans fats. The same study also found that women who ate trans fats were more likely to get type 2 diabetes.

Another study, this one published in a 2007 issue of the journal *Circulation*, included thirty-three thousand women. It found that women with the most trans fats in their blood were three times more likely to get heart disease than women with the lowest amounts of trans fats in their blood. According to Dr. Mozaffarian's 2006 study, eating just a tiny amount of trans fats, as little as 20 to 60 calories worth per day, can greatly increase a person's odds of getting heart disease.

Chapter Four

Getting Trans Fats Out of Your Diet

You may have heard the old saying "Everything in moderation." With trans fats, that's actually untrue. A 2002 report from the Institute of Medicine states that trans fats have a "tolerable upper intake level (UL) of zero." That means there is no amount of trans fat that is safe to eat. Health experts say that because trans fats offer no health benefits and come with a lot of health risks, there isn't any amount worth eating.

Read the Labels

It's hard to avoid a substance that is everywhere you look, but it's not impossible. You just have to start reading labels. Every single "Nutrition Facts" label on the side of a food package lists trans fats. Try to stick to foods that contain 0 grams of trans fats.

This may sound easy, but it's a bit tricky. Some trans fats are carefully hidden. What

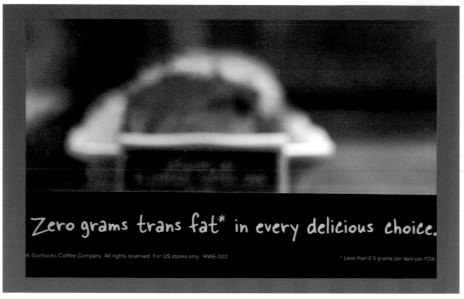

Zero grams trans fat* in every delicious choice.

6 Starbucks Coffee Company. All rights reserved. For US stores only. HWE-002   * Less than 0.5 grams per item per FDA

Read food labels carefully. A package labeled as containing "zero grams trans fat" might not be completely trans fat–free. As the asterisked line in this fast-food restaurant ad explains, the items sold there contain less than 0.5 gram of trans fat, which, per FDA rules, can be listed as trans fat–free.

you think you see may not be what you're actually getting. The FDA requires manufacturers to list trans fats only when their product contains more than 0.5 gram of them. So, a package labeled "fat-free" or "trans fat–free" might contain trans fat.

To know for sure whether or not the food that you're eating contains trans fats, you also have to read the ingredients. Look for words such as "partially hydrogenated vegetable oil," "hydrogenated," or "shortening." These clues will point you to hidden trans fats. The closer to the top of the ingredient list these substances are, the more trans fats the product contains.

In addition, watch out for other unhealthy ingredients listed on the label, such as saturated fat, cholesterol, sodium, and sugar. If you look over on the right side of the label, it lists the "% daily value." Aim for foods that get 5 percent or less of their daily value from these substances. Twenty percent of the daily value is too high—avoid these foods completely.

Knowing how much trans fat is in your food gets a bit harder when you eat out. Some fast-food restaurants now list the nutritional content of their foods, including trans fat, on their Web sites. For those restaurants that don't share that information, you have to ask. Find out what kind of oils they use for cooking and baking. If they use partially hydrogenated vegetable oil or margarine, ask that your food be cooked in olive oil or another trans fat–free vegetable oil. Or, eat somewhere else.

How Much Fat Do You Need?

The FDA says you should get no more than 25 to 35 percent of your daily calories from fat. That includes all kinds of fat. So, if you eat a 2,000-calorie-per-day diet, only about 500 to 700 calories should come from fat. Less than 10 percent, or 200 calories, should come from saturated fat. Get most of your fats from polyunsaturated and monounsaturated sources, such as fish, vegetable oils (flaxseed, olive, peanut, and canola oils), and nuts.

As for trans fat, the FDA hasn't recommended any Daily Reference Value because it says it doesn't have enough information to give an exact amount. In its 2005 Dietary Guidelines, though, the FDA advised that people eat as little of trans-fatty acids as possible. The American Heart Association's 2006 Diet and Lifestyle Recommendations say that even 1 percent of trans fat (2 grams) in your daily diet is too much.

The exception to the rule is trans fats from natural sources. Milk and meat are OK to eat in moderation. Stick to low-fat or skim milk and lean meats—they're the healthiest kinds.

Building a Better Oreo

Since they were introduced in 1912, Oreos have become the classic American cookie. Kids love to separate the chocolate cookies and dunk them in milk, then lick off the creamy filling that's inside. By 2002, people around the world had eaten more than 450 billion Oreo cookies, according to the Kraft Foods, Inc., Web site.

In 2003, British-born lawyer Stephen Joseph sued Kraft to stop it from marketing Oreos to elementary school students in California. Why would anyone want to keep such a childhood favorite away from kids? The trouble was trans fats: Oreos were loaded with them (2.5 grams per three-cookie serving).

Although Joseph later dropped his lawsuit, it did make its mark. In 2004, Kraft announced that it was releasing new kinds of Oreo cookies containing 0 grams of trans fat. Other companies, including Frito-Lay (Doritos, Tostitos, and Cheetos), have also come out with trans fat–free snacks.

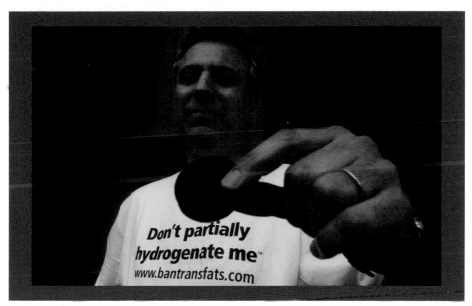

Lawyer Stephen Joseph sued Kraft Foods, Inc., to stop the company from selling Oreos to students in California because of their trans fat content. In part thanks to the lawsuit, Kraft now manufactures trans fat–free Oreos.

Making Better Food Choices

Consumer groups are calling for the food industry to rid trans fats from their food. Until that happens, though, you're in charge of ensuring that trans fats stay out of your diet. In order for you to stay as healthy as possible, your diet should include all of the following:

- Fresh fruits and vegetables
- Whole-grain breads and pastas
- Lean meat, chicken, and fish
- Low-fat dairy products (cheese, yogurt, skim milk)

33

10 Great Questions to Ask

1   What effects will eating trans fats have on my health?

2   How are trans fats different from other types of fats?

3   What kinds of food are made with trans fats?

4   Am I eating too many foods containing trans fats?

5   How much trans fats should I be eating every day?

6   What are the best ways to limit the amount of trans fats in my diet?

7   Do I need to limit other types of fats besides trans fats?

8   How should I read the nutrition label on food packages and on restaurant Web sites?

9   Am I at risk for high cholesterol, high blood pressure, diabetes, or heart disease?

10   What are some other ways that I can stay healthy? For example, how often and for how long should I exercise each week?

- Nuts and seeds
- Unsaturated oils (including olive oil, peanut oil, sesame oil, and sunflower oil)

Limit foods that are high in cholesterol and saturated fat, such as egg yolks, whole milk, and fatty meats. Also cut down on fried foods, as well as cookies and other baked goods. Watch your portion sizes as well. One serving of microwave popcorn may contain less than a gram of trans fat, but if you eat an entire bowl, you'll be consuming far more than that!

To lower the amount of trans fats in your diet, try switching some of the foods you usually eat to these healthier options:

Instead of . . .	Try . . .
Margarine	Olive oil
A doughnut	A whole-wheat bagel
Apple pie	Strawberries with fat-free whipped topping
French fries	A side salad with light dressing
Crackers	Nuts
Potato chips	Fat-free pretzels

Eating Healthy at School

Your quest for healthy eating doesn't end when the school bell rings. You need to be just as conscious of what you eat in the cafeteria as you do at home and in restaurants. Many schools are offering healthier choices.

They're replacing pizza and burgers with salads and sandwiches. They're switching from sodas to water and fruit juice, and they're ditching cookies and cakes.

If your school isn't offering healthy options, either bring your lunch from home or be more selective about your choices. Have a side salad with your slice of pizza. (Just remember to limit the salad dressing.) Order your turkey sandwich on whole-wheat bread instead of white. Eat an apple or nonfat yogurt instead of ice cream for dessert. When you do eat unhealthy snacks, don't eat them every day and be sure to watch your portions. Remember that you only have one body. It's up to you to treat it right if you want to look and feel your best!

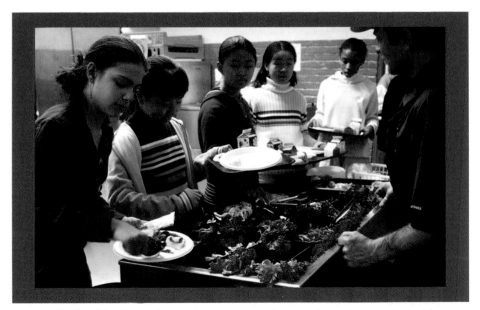

Among the healthy lunch items these Connecticut students have selected in their school cafeteria are fruit and vegetables. Making healthy food choices is important both at home and at school.

Glossary

arteries Vessels that carry blood from the heart to the rest of the body.

asthma A condition in which air passages become narrowed or blocked, making it difficult to breathe.

cholesterol A fatlike substance found in certain foods that is carried through the blood. Low-density lipoprotein (LDL) cholesterol is the "bad" type of cholesterol because it can build up in arteries and block blood flow. High-density lipoprotein (HDL) cholesterol is the "good" type because it helps remove excess cholesterol from the body.

cis fatty acid A type of unsaturated fatty acid in which the hydrogen atoms are on the same side of the fatty acid chain.

fatty acid Chemical compound that makes up fats. A fatty acid consists of a chain of carbon and hydrogen atoms.

heart attack A condition in which blood flow through an artery to the heart is blocked. The lack of blood causes the heart muscle to die.

heart disease Damage to the heart and blood vessels that affects the ability of the heart to work as well as it should.

hydrogenation The process of adding hydrogen to liquid vegetable oil to produce a more solid and stable (but unhealthier) kind of fat.

insulin A hormone that helps regulate the amount of sugar in the blood and helps the cells of the body use that sugar for energy.

lipoprotein (a) A chemical compound made up of fat and protein that carries cholesterol in the blood.

monounsaturated fat A type of unsaturated fat in which there is one double-bonded carbon atom in the fatty acid chain.

omega-3 fatty acid A type of fatty acid found in fish, flax seeds, and canola oil that is believed to protect the heart.

polyunsaturated fat A type of unsaturated fat in which there is more than one double-bonded carbon atom in the fatty acid chain.

saturated fat An unhealthy type of fat found in animal products (meat, whole milk), in which a hydrogen atom is connected to every single carbon atom on the fatty acid chain.

sleep apnea A condition in which one's breathing is interrupted many times while asleep. It can be caused by an obstruction, such as enlarged tonsils, in the passageway connecting the throat and nose. Being overweight can affect the development of sleep apnea.

stroke A condition that occurs when a blockage cuts off blood flow to the brain. Affected parts of the brain can die, leading to slurred speech, loss of movement, and death.

trans fat An unhealthy type of fat found in cookies, pies, and french fries. Most trans fats come from a process called hydrogenation.

triglyceride A type of fat that is transported in the blood. Raised levels of triglycerides may lead to heart disease.

tumor An abnormal growth of tissue that can be cancerous.

type 2 diabetes A disease that occurs when the body can no longer use insulin properly. It is more common in people who are overweight.

unsaturated fat A type of fat in which hydrogen is not attached to every carbon atom in the fatty acid chain.

For More Information

Action for Healthy Kids
4711 West Golf Road, Suite 625
Skokie, IL 60076
(800) 416-5136
Web site: http://www.actionforhealthykids.org
This group helps kids eat better and become more active.

American Dietetic Association
120 South Riverside Plaza, Suite 2000
Chicago, IL 60606-6995
(800) 877-1600
Web site: http://www.eatright.org
The American Dietetic Association is the biggest group
    of food and nutrition experts in the country. It helps
    people eat healthier and prevent obesity.

American Heart Association
National Center
7272 Greenville Avenue
Dallas, TX 75231
(800) 242-8721
Web site: http://www.americanheart.org
The American Heart Association conducts research
    and educates the public to prevent heart disease
    and stroke.

Canadian Council of Food and Nutrition
2810 Matheson Boulevard East, 1st Floor
Mississauga, ON L4W 4X7
Canada
(905) 625-5746
Web site: http://www.ccfn.ca
This Canadian organization is made up of health experts
    who teach the public about food and nutrition issues.

Center for Food Safety & Applied Nutrition
U.S. Food and Drug Administration
5100 Paint Branch Parkway
College Park, MD 20740-3835
(888) 463-6332
Web site: http://www.cfsan.fda.gov
This branch of the Food and Drug Administration
    regulates the safety of food products. It also educates
    consumers about nutritional health.

Dietitians of Canada
480 University Avenue, Suite 604
Toronto, ON M5G 1V2
Canada
(416) 596-0857
Web site: http://www.dietitians.ca
This group of dietitians provides food and nutrition
    advice to people living in Canada.

MyPyramid.gov
USDA Center for Nutrition Policy and Promotion

41

3101 Park Center Drive, Room 1034
Alexandria, VA 22302-1594
(888) 779-7264
Web site: http://www.mypyramid.gov
The U.S. Department of Agriculture's MyPyramid.gov
   site offers a personal eating plan with recommendations for the healthy kinds of food and amounts that
   are best for your body type and lifestyle.

Web Sites

Due to the changing nature of Internet links, Rosen
Publishing has developed an online list of Web sites
related to the subject of this book. This site is updated
regularly. Please use this link to access the list:

http://www.rosenlinks.com/wyf/trfa

For Further Reading

Coons, Steve, and Kevin Murdoch. *The Lifestyle Journey Program*. Newmarket, ON: Ideas for People, Inc., 2002.

Figtree, Dale. *Eat Smarter: The Smarter Choice for Healthier Kids*. El Monte, CA: ZHealth Books, 2006.

Haduch, Bill, and Rick Stromoski. *Food Rules! The Stuff You Munch, Its Crunch, Its Punch, and Why You Sometimes Lose Your Lunch*. New York, NY: Puffin Books, 2001.

Harmon, Daniel E. *Obesity* (Coping in a Changing World). New York, NY: Rosen Publishing, 2007.

Jukes, Mavis, and Lilian Wai-Yin Cheung. *Be Healthy! It's a Girl Thing: Food, Fitness, and Feeling Great*. New York, NY: Crown Publishers, 2003.

Levin, Judith. *Frequently Asked Questions About Diabetes* (FAQ: Teen Life). New York, NY: Rosen Publishing, 2007.

Nardo, Don. *Understanding Issues—Eating Disorders*. Farmington Hills, MI: KidHaven Press, 2003.

Platkin, Charles. *Lighten Up*. New York, NY: Penguin Young Readers Group, 2005.

Schlosser, Eric, and Charles Wilson. *Chew on This: Everything You Don't Want to Know About Fast Food*. New York, NY: Houghton-Mifflin, 2006.

Bibliography

American Heart Association. "Cardiovascular Disease Statistics." Retrieved May 1, 2007 (http://www. americanheart.org/presenter.jhtml?identifier = 4478).

American Heart Association. "Diet and Lifestyle Recommendations Revision 2006." *Circulation*, Vol. 114, July 4, 2006, pp. 82–96.

Bowman, Shanthy A., Steven L. Gortmaker, Cara B. Ebbeling, Mark A. Pereira, and David S. Ludwig. "Effects of Fast-Food Consumption on Energy Intake and Diet Quality Among Children in a National Household Survey." *Pediatrics*, Vol. 113, No. 1, January 2004, pp. 112–118.

Centers for Disease Control and Prevention. "Overweight and Obesity." August 26, 2006. Retrieved May 1, 2007 (http://www.cdc.gov/ nccdphp/dnpa/obesity/index.htm).

Centers for Disease Control and Prevention, National Center for Health Statistics. "Overweight." Retrieved May 1, 2007 (http://www.cdc.gov/nchs/fastats/ overwt.htm).

Gosline, Anna. "Why Fast Foods Are Bad, Even in Moderation." NewScientist.com, June 12, 2006. Retrieved September 17, 2007 (http://www. newscientist.com/article/dn9318.html).

Harrison, Kristen, and Amy L. Markse. "Nutritional Content of Foods Advertised During the Television Programs Children Watch Most." *American Journal of Public Health*, Vol. 95, No. 9, September 2005, pp. 1,568–1,574.

Institute of Medicine. *Letter Report on Dietary Reference Intakes for Trans Fatty Acids*. 2002. Retrieved May 11, 2007 (http://www.iom.edu/Object.File/Master/13/083/TransFattyAcids.pdf).

Kher, Unmesh. "Target: Trans Fats." *Time*, Vol. 166, October 24, 2005, pp. 53–54.

Mozaffarian, Dariush, Martijn B. Katan, Alberto Ascherio, Meir J. Stampfer, and Walter C. Willett. "Trans Fatty Acids and Cardiovascular Disease." *New England Journal of Medicine*, Vol. 354, April 13, 2006, pp. 1,601–1,613.

Shaw, Judith. *Trans Fats: The Hidden Killer in Our Food.* New York, NY: Pocket Books, 2004.

Singer, D. J., and J. L. Singer, eds. *The Handbook of Children and Media.* Thousand Oaks, CA: Sage, 2001.

Squires, Sally. "Panel Urges Schools to Replace Junk Foods." *Washington Post*, April 26, 2007, p. A03.

Stender, Steen, Jørn Dyerberg, and Arne Astrup. "High Levels of Industrially Produced Trans Fat in Popular Fast Food." *New England Journal of Medicine*, Vol. 354, April 13, 2006, pp. 1,650–1,652.

Sun, Qi, Jing Ma, Hannia Campos, Susan E. Hankinson, JoAnn E. Manson, Meir J. Stampfer, Kathryn M. Rexrode, Walter C. Willett, and Frank B. Hu. "A

Prospective Study of Trans Fatty Acids in Erythrocytes and Risk of Coronary Heart Disease." *Circulation*, Vol. 115, April 10, 2007, pp. 1,858–1,865.

USDA Dietary Guidelines 2005. January 12, 2005. Retrieved March 25, 2007 (http://www.health.gov/ dietaryguidelines/dga2005/document/html/ executivesummary.htm).

U.S. Department of Health and Human Services. The President's Council on Physical Fitness and Sports. "Physical Activity Facts." January 18, 2007. Retrieved May 5, 2007 (http://www.fitness.gov/resources_ factsheet.htm).

U.S. Food and Drug Administration. "Questions and Answers About Trans Fat Nutrition Labeling." January 1, 2006. Retrieved April 17, 2007 (http:// www.cfsan.fda.gov/~ dms/qatrans2.html).

U.S. Food and Drug Administration. "Revealing Trans Fats." FDA Consumer, September–October 2003. Retrieved March 26, 2007 (http://www.fda.gov/ FDAC/features/2003/503_fats.html).

U.S. Food and Drug Administration. "Trans Fat Now Listed with Saturated Fat and Cholesterol on the Nutrition Facts Label." January 1, 2006. Retrieved April 11, 2007 (http://www.cfsan.fda.gov/~ dms/ transfat.html).

Willett, W. C. "Intake of Trans Fatty Acids and Risk of Coronary Heart Disease Among Women." *The Lancet*, Vol. 341, March 6, 1993, pp. 581–585.

Index

About the Author

Stephanie Watson is a writer and editor based in Atlanta, Georgia. She has written or contributed to more than a dozen health and science books, including *Endometriosis*, *Encyclopedia of the Human Body: The Endocrine System*, *The Mechanisms of Genetics: An Anthology of Current Thought*, and *Science and Its Times*. Her work has also been featured on several health and wellness Web sites, including Rosen Publishing's Teen Health and Wellness database, for which she contributed several entries about eating disorders.

Photo Credits

Cover (doughnuts) © www.istockphoto.com/Cole Vineyard, (chicken, pie) © www.istockphoto.com/Jack Puccio, (fries) © www.istockphoto.com/Andrew Manley, (candy) © www.istockphoto.com/Emre YILDIZ; p. 5 © Kevin Summers/Stone/Getty Images; p. 14 © Mary Evans Picture Library/The Image Works; pp. 17, 22 © AP Images; p. 19 © Tim Boyle/Getty Images; p. 25 © Robin Lazarus/Custom Medical Stock Photo; p. 28 © Mario Tama/Getty Images; p. 30 © KC Alfred/San Diego Union Tribune/Zuma Press; p. 33 © Wimborne/Reuters/Landov; p. 36 © Peter Hvizdak/The Image Works.

Designer: Tahara Anderson; **Editor:** Kathy Kuhtz Campbell
Photo Researcher: Amy Feinberg